This book belongs to:

_____

_____

MEDICAL NOTES ON CANNABIS
(aka MARIJUANA)
FROM 1887

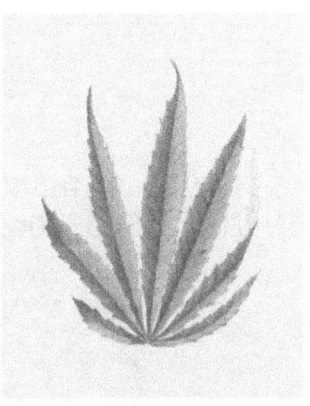

by
Charles F. Millspaugh, M.D.

ISBN-13: 978-1546540427
ISBN-10: 1546540423

These medical notes were
extracted word for word
from the old book,
"American Medicinal Plants
An Illustrated And Descriptive Guide
To The American Plants
Used As Homeopathic Remedies:
Their History, Preparation,
Chemistry, And
Physiological Effects".
Written by
Charles F. Millspaugh, M.D.
and published in 1887
by Boericke & Tafel.

N. ORD. URTICACEÆ.
TRIBE. – CANNABINEÆ.
GENUS. – CANNABIS,[1 see page 24]
        TOURN.
SEX. SYST. – DIŒCIA PENTANDRIA.

CANNABIS.
HEMP.

SYN. – CANNABIS SATIVA, LINN.;
CANNABIS INDICA, LAM.
COM. NAMES. – INDIAN HEMP;
(FR.) CHANVRE; (GER.) HANF.

A TINCTURE OF THE TOPS OF
AMERICAN-GROWN CANNABIS
SATIVA, LINN.

Description. — This tall,
roughish annual, usually grows
from 3 to 10 feet high. *Stem* erect,
striate, roughish, ligneous at the
base, simple or sparingly branched;
inner bark tough and fibrous.

Leaves digitately-compound, the lower opposite, the upper alternate; *leaflets* 3-5-7, linear-lanceolate, coarsely and sharply serrate, attenuate at both ends; finely scabrous, and dark-green above, pale and downy beneath; *petioles* long, slender, and scabrous; *stipules* linear, acute. *In-florescence* diœcious. *Sterile flowers* in axillary compound racemes, or panicles; *sepals* 5, nearly separate, reflexed-spreading, nearly equal, oblong and downy; *stamens* 5, opposite the segments of the calyx; *filaments* short, drooping, not inflexed in the bud; *anthers* large, pendulous, 2-celled. *Fertile flowers* in axillary, spiked clusters, leafy below; *flowers* 1-bracted and sessile; *calyx* of a single, 5-veined, hirsute sepal, enlarging and cordate at the base, acute at the apex; *ovary* 1-celled; *ovule* single, erect, orthotropous;

style not evident; *stigmas* 2, elongated, hairy, protruding far beyond the perianth. *Fruit* a glandular achenium, enwrapped by the persistent sepal; *pericarp* membranaceous, indehiscent, but easily separable by pressure into two valves. *Seed* ovoid, smooth, brown, and veiny; *embryo* simply curved; *albumen* slight, oleaginous.

History and Habitat. — This native of the temperate portions of Asia — a plant of ancient cultivation — grows readily in this country, in waste places and cultivated grounds, where the cleanings of bird cages have found their way. It thrives well, [2 see page 24] blossoming in July and August.

The plant in its travels westward is supposed to have reached Italy during the Roman period, from whence it has spread in all temperate regions of the globe. It does not seem to have been known to the ancient Egyptians as having narcotic properties. Herodotus terms the plant Κάνναβις nuepos; stating that the Thracians made a kind of cloth of it. The seeds were also thrown upon red-hot stones, and their perfumed vapor, so obtained, used for a fume bath, which excited from those enjoying it, cries of exultation. Dr. Royle considers it the Nepenthes of Homer, "the assuager of grief," given by Helen to Telemachus in honor of Menelaus; she is said to have received the plant from an Egyptian woman of Thebes. Dioscorides recommends the herb in the form of a cataplasm for inflammations, and to discuss tumors. Paulus Ægineta says the seeds are carminative and desiccative, and the juice of the fresh plant useful for pain and obstructions of the ears. In India, the plant is known by names which translated mean, "Grass of Fakirs", "Leaf of Delusion", "Increaser of Pleasure", "Exciter of Desire", "Laughter Mover", and "Cementer of Friendship."

The true Indian Hemp, *i.e.*, that which contains to the fullest extent the narcotic properties of the herb, grows at altitudes of 6,000 feet and over, principally in the Himalayas above Calcutta, and in Thibet. These plants differ in nowise botanically from those that grow at lower levels, but medically the variation is wide. It is certainly admissible here to mention the products of the more active form which, for convenience, we will retain as *Cannabis Indica*. The principal commercial form of the Indian plant is called *Gunjah*,

Ganja, or in England *Guaza*. It is this form that reaches the American markets through London, and from which our tincture of *C. Indica* should be made. It consists, according to a fine specimen kindly given us by Shifflein & Co., of New York, of the dried, flowering tops, compressed into small, ovoid masses, cohering by the natural resin contained, and composed of small floral leaves, female flowers, and undeveloped seed. Each separate mass exhales a small portion of the stemlet upon which it grew, and exhales to a high degree the odor peculiar to the plant. This *Gunja* yields an excellent extract, which, when at a temperature of 65°F., is thick, and only runs when held a long time at a sharp angle; it is of so dark a green color as to appear jet black; has a strongly narcotic, peculiar, and not unpleasant odor; is very adhesive, insoluble in water, and fully soluble in alcohol, its solution having a brilliant green color. When placed upon the tongue no taste is at first noticed on account of its very slow solubility in the natural secretions of the mouth, but after a few moments the taste is a counterpart of the odor, and when the solution reaches the base of the tongue an agreeable bitter is notable. This extract was formerly used for our tincture. Other forms of the plant sold in India and Arabia are, *a.* Bhang, Subjee, or Sidhee, which consists of the dried leaves broken into coarse powder with which are intermixed a few seeds. This form is used for smoking, and is the narcotic ingredient of the confection called *Majun. β. Charas*, or *Churrus*, consisting of the natural resin of the tops and leaves, mixed with bits of the plant and much dirt. This form is usually procured by natives who pass among the plants, wearing a leathern apron to which the resin adheres; in the mean time the plant tops are rubbed with their hands, and afterward the hands and aprons scraped to gather the product, *y. Hashisch*, *Hashish*, or *Hashash*. These are the Arabian names for hemp. The product consists of the dried flowering tops gathered before the fruits are formed. The famous heretical sect of Mohammedans, who, by murderous attacks upon the Crusaders, struck their hearts with terror, derived their name *Hashashin* from the drug, and from that our word *assassin* is derived, *ð. Hemp*. This textile is produced principally by those plants whose narcotic powers are least marked; those that grow in the lower altitudes producing the best article. This product is made into ropes and coarse cloths, *ε. Hemp Seed*. The seeds of this plant are considered fattening, and egg-producing when fed to birds. Cage-birds are particularly fond of them, but on account of their limited chances for exercise only a few *per diem* are usually allowed them. *ζ. Oil of Hemp Seed*. The seeds yield about 25 per cent, of their weight of a limpid, almost colorless oil, that makes a fine burning-fluid, and is used in the arts for mixing colors, and as a varnish.

In general practice the drug is used wherever an anodyne, hypnotic, or antispasmodic is judged necessary; the various diseases where it proves effectual are hardly mentionable, as the benefit is almost always homœopathic, therefore, each disease should be individualized. Surgical tetanus, gonorrhœa, leucorrhœa, inflammation of the mucous membranes of the bladder and urethra, dysuria, delirium, and melancholia may be, however, mentioned as the diseases in which our Old School brothers usually get the most decided effects from this drug.

Cannabis Americana, *i.e.* the tops of American-grown plants, are officinal in the U.S. Ph. The plant is mentioned in the Eclectic Dispensatory, but no preparation is given.

Part Used And Preparation. — The fresh flowering tops of the American-grown plants, both male and female, are treated as directed under Celtis. The tincture, after straining and filtering, is opaque; has an herbaceous odor; a sweetish mucoid taste, followed by slight bitterness; and an acid reaction. The two tinctures of this plant may be compared as follows:

Cannabis Sativa.

Americana.
Domestic Growth.
Tincture.

Appearance, in bulk, deep opaque brown.

Twenty drops in a drachm of alcohol give an orange-brown color by transmitted light.

Ten drops in two drachms of water quickly show the difference in the amount of resin.

This tincture shows only slight opalescence; while

In this tincture the peculiar pungent and heavy narcotic odor of *Gunja* is faintly, if at all, noticeable.

Indica.
Indian Growth at 6,000 Feet.
Tincture.

Deep opaque greenish-brown.

A slight greenish tinge only is noticeable; the two solutions nearly correspond.

This gives a completely opaque, heavy, dirty cream-colored mass.

In this the odor is plainly distinguishable.

As the narcotic power of the drug lies mostly in the resin of the plant, the activity of the two states of the plant is readily understood by the above comparison, simple as it is.

Chemical Constituents. — As far as I can determine, the

American plant has not been analyzed, but as it at least contains a small amount of the resinoid principle of the Indian plant, it may be well to glance at the chemistry of Gunja, as it stands at this date. There is great uncertainty concerning the active principle of this drug, as the *Cannabin* of the Smiths fails, so far, to answer, at the hands of other chemists, to the characteristics claimed for it by them. Worden and Waddle find the nicotia-like alkaloid of Preobraschersky, but in their hands it proves inert; and, though Siebold and Bradbury found a volatile alkaloid (*Cannabinine*), they claim that it is unlike nicotia, though they have not tested its action upon animals. Merck isolated a glucoside, which he combines with tannin and calls *Cannabin Tannin*, and from which Bombelon obtained a body he terms *Cannabinum*; this tannin compound often proves inert. Matthew Hay reports an alkaloid, forming in acicular crystals, and having a tetanic action upon frogs, which he calls *Tetano-Cannabin*, and considers as a secondary principle.[3 see page 24] This is about the condition of the chemistry of this drug today; which the following digest will farther explain:

Cannabin. — This body, extracted from Gunja, by Messrs. T. and H. Smith,[4 see page 24] and considered much purer than Gastinel's *Hashascin*, results as a brown, amorphous, solid resin, which burns with a bright flame, leaving no ash, and is soluble in alcohol and ether. It is claimed, by its discoverers, to be very potent, two-thirds of a grain proving decidedly narcotic, and one grain causing complete intoxication. Personne claims that the activity of this body is due to the volatile oil, but his method of extracting the body was sufficient to render it inert, rendering his claim, therefore, inadmissible. Bolas and Francis[5 see page 24] obtained from this body:

Oxycannabin, $C_{20}H_{20}N_2O_7$, which resulted in large, neutral prisms, from its solution in methylic alcohol. These crystals melt at 176° (348.8°F.), and evaporate without decomposition. Fückiger failed to obtain this body from purified resin of Charas.[6 see page 24]

Oil of Cannabis. — This volatile, pale yellow oil, was discovered in the tops by Personne, [7 see page 24&25] who claimed it to be the active principle of the plant, and to cause, in those who inhaled its effluvium, shuddering, and

desire for locomotion, followed by prostration and sometimes syncope. Bolig obtained this oil from the fresh tops of the Arabian plant, and found its effects to be similar to those claimed for it by Personne, and further stated that it contained oxygen. Personne succeeded in separating the oil into two hydrocarbons: *Cannabine*, $C_{18}H_{20}$, and
Cannabine Hydride, $C_{18}H_{22}$, the latter being a solid composed of platy crystals.

Other unessential bodies have been determined, to none of which the activity of the drug can be assigned.

Physiological Action. — Carefully excluding, as far as possible, symptoms that may have arisen from the Indian product, the following will give some idea of the action of the herb of low altitudes, collated from the experiments of Drs. Schreter, Knorre, Wibmer, Wirk, and Lembke with the tincture, in doses of from 5 to 70 drops, and the infusion:[8 see page 25] Depression and absentmindedness; confusion, vertigo, and congestion, followed by cephalalgia; earache; toothache; dryness of the mouth, throat, and lips; loss of appetite; nausea, and vomiting after coffee; slight inflammation of the meatus urinarius, and diminished urine; sexual excitement without desire; oppression of the chest, and palpitation of the heart; weakness of the limbs; itching of the skin; and dreaminess during sleep.

References:

[1] *Κάνναβις, Kannabis*; an Oriental name of unknown meaning, probably, however, derived from the Arabian name of the plant *ganeb*.

[2] A thrifty female plant, nine feet high, grew last year in a farm-house yard near Binghamton; and several of both sexes, fully seven feet, at Union, N.Y.

[3] Am. Four. Phar., 1885, 264; from Phar. Four, and Trans., 1885, 574.

[4] Phar. Four., 1847, 171.

[5] Chem. News, 1871, 77.

[6] Pharmacographia, 549.

[7] Four. de Phar., 1857, 48;

Medical Notes On Cannabis
(aka Marijuana) From 1887

Canstatt's *Fahres.*, 1857, 28.

[8] Allen, *Ency.*, 2, 492, *et seq.*

Description of Plate.

Drawn from plants growing at Union, N.Y., July 26th, 1886.

1. A portion of male inflorescence.
2. Sterile flower.
3. A portion of female inflorescence.
4. Female flowers.
5. Male flower-bud.
6, 7, 8. Stamens.
9. Female flower.
10. Calyx of female flower.
11. Ovary.
12. Section of ovary.
13. Styles.
14, 15, 16. Fruit.
17, 18, 19. Seed.
20. Longitudinal section } of a seed.
21. Horizontal section } of a seed.
22. Embryo.
        (2 and 4-22 enlarged.)

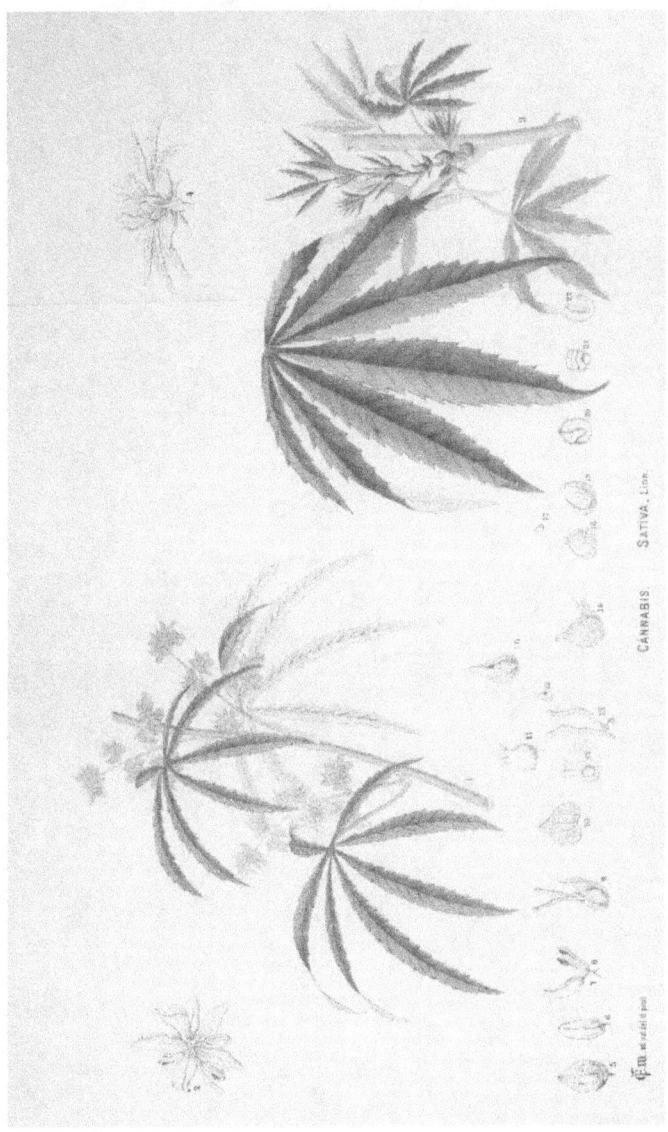